Anti-Inflammatory Diet

A Nutritionist's Guide to Reduce Inflammation Naturally - Calm Hashimoto's, Crohn's, IBS & Other Autoimmune Disorders

SIMON KELLER

© Copyright 2018 – (Simon Keller) **All rights reserved.**

The contents of this book may not be reproduced, duplicated or transmitted without direct written permission from the author. Under no circumstances will any legal responsibility or blame be held against the publisher for any reparation, damages, or monetary loss due to the information herein, either directly or indirectly.

Legal Notice:

This book is copyright protected. This is only for personal use. You cannot amend, distribute, sell, use, quote or paraphrase any part or the content within this book without the consent of the author.

Disclaimer Notice:

Please note the information contained within this document is for educational and entertainment purposes only. Every attempt has been made to provide accurate, up to date and reliable complete information. No warranties of any kind are expressed or implied. Readers acknowledge that the author is not engaging in the rendering of legal, financial, medical or professional advice. The content of this book has been derived from various sources. Please consult a licensed professional before attempting any techniques outlined in this book.

By reading this document, the reader agrees that under no circumstances is the author responsible for any losses, direct or indirect, which are incurred as a result of the use of information contained within this document, including, but not limited to, — errors, omissions, or inaccuracies.

TABLE OF CONTENTS

Introduction 1

My Credentials 5

Part 1: A Background & Overview of Inflammation 9

Chapter 1: Understanding Acute vs Chronic Inflammation 11

Chapter 2: Symptoms, Causes & Conditions 15

Chapter 3: How to Seek the Correct Medical Help (if Needed) 21

Part 2: Practical Ways to Reduce Inflammation in the Body - Everyday Tips & Eating Plans 27

Chapter 4: Lifestyle Interventions to Reduce
Inflammation Naturally 29

Chapter 5: Remember Food is Thy Medicine 37

Chapter 6: A Word on Pesticides - Clean Fifteen vs Dirty Dozen 41

Chapter 7: Removing Gluten & Diary - A Game Changer 47

Chapter 8: Other Food Groups to Include & Avoid 53

Chapter 9: Meal Plans - Vegan, Paleo & Mediterranean Options 63

Summary 71

Conclusion 77

Bonus Chapter 79

INTRODUCTION

It's important to point out that inflammation is a natural occurrence within the body. It's a cleansing mechanism which flushes away toxins and impurities. It's the first stage in the healing process which initiates other autoimmune activities to kick into gear.

There is however a flip side to this situation. When inflammation starts to become chronic, enduring and out of control. This is when things start to become a problem. If left unchecked, it will stimulate an ever increasing number of immune cells to become recruited into a never ending battle to stave off serious illness and disease.

In the most extreme cases, this inflammatory response can begin to contribute to the problem, as healthy tissue starts to come under fire. The body's immune system turns against itself. This is when the most chronic of autoimmune diseases can arise.

Unfortunately this is a widespread problem we face across the world today, especially in Western nations who have developed very poor eating and lifestyle habits. We are combining a mixture of poor nutrition, physical inactivity, environmental toxins, excessive pharmaceutical medications, on top of stressful jobs and a lack of adequate sleep.

This is a recipe for disaster for the immune system. It's a cocktail of components which perfectly induce and exacerbate inflammation causing processes within the body. In reality, this is what the general population is fighting against. Not necessarily the end forms of these debilitating disorders just yet. But a dampening of inflammatory fires on a daily basis, which can lead to bigger issues if allowed to persist.

So my aim for this edition in the diet and detox series is to once again shed some light on the factors which promote these problems, as well as educate you on the main health considerations caused by the negative side of inflammation.

But more importantly, how best to prepare for and deal with these consequences. To provide the practical steps you can take each day to halt chronic inflammation in its tracks. To reverse the symptoms and conditions you may be experiencing from existing poor lifestyle choices.

In that sense, this should be a starting point. You should always be consulting your local GP and be under the guidance of health care professionals, when undertaking any significant dietary changes in your life. Especially if you believe you are suffering from chronic inflammation or autoimmune disorders already.

Dietary and lifestyle interventions are always going to be the best long term preventative measures in my opinion though. Getting back to eating the foods our body's were designed to consume, will naturally re-set any imbalances in the system. It will calm the irritations you may be experiencing from aggravating your cells and tissues with these foreign food sources. So get ready to give this a try, you'll thank yourself in the long run.

MY CREDENTIALS

Before we get into the specifics of an anti-inflammatory diet, it's always a good idea for me to explain exactly who I am, and why you should bother listening to me in the first place. Yes I have an undergraduate degree in anatomy/physiology from the University of Birmingham in the UK.

However, my main focus over the past 10 years has been on the practical implications of human performance. I now focus much more on the results of these principles in the real world, compared to my previous life of studying endless research papers on the academic side of the subject.

This includes everything from human movement to dietary considerations. What set of variables is most optimal for both myself, and the clients I now coach and mentor within my specialized training and wellness complex here in London.

Not everyone is a carbon copy of each other, however there is a great deal of overlap when it comes to human physiology. Discounting some minor age, gender and hereditary considerations, we are all working with pretty much the same metabolic machinery. You just need to know how to get the most from it.

So why am I such an expert on inflammation causing conditions? As I mentioned, I studied a wide range of topics within the field of cardiovascular/respiratory physiology and biochemistry whilst at university. This formed my base understanding of these subjects and how they fit together within a holistic sense.

Although I have since put these academic theories and principles to the test in the real world. To really see what works and what doesn't with regards to completing the health and fitness puzzle.

Diet and lifestyle considerations are obviously major factors which play into this. Getting your food right and reducing your exposure to excessive stress and outside pollutants, is key to protecting the body from unwanted inflammation.

I'm continually monitoring my clients for signs chronic autoimmune responses, as this will have such a detrimental impact on their overall health, let alone fitness levels if left unmanged. In this sense, I oversee everything from devising peoples workout routines to adjusting their eating plans in order to achieve these goals. To also provide some motivational and psychological guidance along the way.

I believe a 360 degree approach to human performance works best. Creating a work life balance is how you garner optimal results, as everything is then ultimately working in harmony. Of course this goes out of kilter for all of us at one time or another, but hopefully you will now have some better information on how to get yourself back on track if and when you do fall off the horse.

The following chapters will layout the groundwork for doing this. The theories behind what is causing inflammation in the first place, and how you can best implement the practical measures to downplay these negative effects in your own life. To calm the body and return it to an optimal state once again!

PART 1: A BACKGROUND & OVERVIEW OF INFLAMMATION

CHAPTER 1: UNDERSTANDING ACUTE VS CHRONIC INFLAMMATION

Back in 2008 I lived down under in Australia for two years, Melbourne to be exact. I was spending some time in a new environment with some of the sports teams in the city. Predominantly with the professional Australian Rules Football teams or "Auzzie Rules" clubs as the locals refer to them.

However, during this time there were some of the worst forest fires in recorded history, which raged within the outer suburbs of Victoria, the South Eastern State. Summer times in Melbourne were hot, like really hot. I recall it getting up to 52 degrees Celsius (125 degrees Fahrenheit) on a couple of days, and the city pretty much ground to a halt.

I'm used to road closures and sports events being shut down due to bad weather back in the UK. But always due to the cold, either freezing or snowy conditions within the winter time. But in Melbourne it was the opposite. The incredible dry heat prevented most people from leaving the house, let alone going to work or exercising that day. The roads even started to melt in some districts!

But this was nothing compared to what was going on in the surrounding rural area's. Wildfires were sparked and ravaged entire counties within days, sometimes hours. I was told that smaller and more controlled fires were actually very common. They were beneficial and intentional in some cases, as they would clear the area of old and dead bush-lands ready for new plant and wildlife to grow in its place.

However, the fires which raged that year were far more sinister than this. They were uncontrollable and enduring waves of heat which consumed pretty much anything in their path. Entire towns were swept up in the crossfire. Residential houses, office buildings and other infrastructure all gone before fire brigade crews could even make a dent in the fires progress.

It reminds me very much of the situation which goes on inside of our bodies with regards to inflammation. There is a fine line between a short and sharp healthy dose, and an out of control blaze which causes far more damage than good. It's beneficial to differentiate between these two instances and take a look at where we should draw the line.

Acute Inflammation

As I mentioned within the introduction to this book. Inflammation is an everyday occurrence within the body. Acute inflammation is normal, it's local and its positive for the most part. If you've ever cut a finger or bruised your leg, than you've experienced this type of inflammation.

In these instances a sensitive alarm system is triggered within the body which works to quickly activate immune system responses. The affected cells can detect the infection or viral threat, and request the necessary reinforcements to diffuse the attack. Surveillance cells will send messengers such as cytokines and adipokines in order to recruit sufficient white blood cells to fight the trauma.

This will not only neutralize harmful toxins and pathogens, but simultaneously signal other pathways to supply the needed oxygen and nutrients to the damaged area, in order for recovery to begin. It's a desirable response to injury or infection within the body. It's a protective short-lived measure designed to soak up harmful compounds by deploying the appropriate anti-bodies, and provide the adequate building blocks for tissue rebuilding and repair.

Chronic Inflammation

Chronic inflammation on the other hand is the opposite. It's widespread, enduring and sadly more prevalent in society than it needs to be. It saps energy and drags those down who develop it. If it's allowed to persist, the immune system will be unable to function properly. Leading onto many debilitative illness and conditions we suffer today.

If the original source of the inflammation can't be tamed, than this irritation can continue to wreak havoc within the body. If the acute inflammation response isn't calibrated correctly, then it can overspill and direct intense immune system attacks on otherwise healthy cells and tissues. This will in turn lead onto a number of autoimmune diseases if we are not careful.

Essentially the autoimmune response goes out of kilter, it becomes unbalanced. It initiates an over exaggerated inflammatory response within the body. The system starts to interpret otherwise neutral cells as harmful, such as skeletal muscle tissue or bone cartilage. It begins to turn the body's own defence mechanisms against itself harming the host in the process.

Of course you can expect some collateral damage in a successful acute inflammation clear-up. But if this response fails to back off in a timely manner, a normal inflammation response can turn into the problem itself. It's the equivalent of using a bucket of water to put out the candles on a birthday cake. It can produce a disease like state such as severe allergies and Lupus if allowed to persist.

The following chapter will explore some of the most prevalent and harmful of these conditions. What are the symptoms you should be looking out for, as well as how they develop in the first place.

CHAPTER 2: SYMPTOMS, CAUSES & CONDITIONS

"Inflammation is a hot topic in medicine. It appears connected to almost every known chronic disease"

(Mark Hyman MD)

Symptoms

There are a number of signs that a person may be experiencing excessive and chronic inflammation within the body. Some are reasonably easy to spot, others are more difficult to detect. The more obvious of these symptoms include:

- Swelling & Bloating
- Soreness & Pain
- Redness & Overheating
- Persistent Headaches

These are the red flags which should encourage you to visit the doctor and get a second opinion on your condition. They will be able to perform tests for the more difficult to spot markers of chronic inflammation such as C-Reactive Protein and Cortisol levels within the bloodstream. More on this within the following chapter regarding medical guidance.

Causes

What isn't in doubt is the fact that genes & hereditary factors play a large role in determining some of the common conditions of chronic inflammation. In recent years many genome sequencing studies have been performed in an attempt to pinpoint the exact causes of these ailments. It has been found that there is significant overlap with regards to the markers of inflammation associated with illnesses such as Crohn's disease and other hereditary conditions such as type 1 diabetes.

However, there is still some way to go in terms of isolating these genes and preventing the body from expressing their negative effects. Knowing this, I believe it to be wise to focus on the things we can affect I.e. the environmental factors within our control. The lifestyle and dietary choices we can choose to make throughout the day, which certainly play their part in terms of the extent and severity of these genetic expressions.

I touched upon these within the opening remarks to this book. Chronic inflammation can be caused an exacerbated by a number of the external factors which include:

- Poor Diet

- Inadequate Exercise

- Environmental Pollutants
- Overuse of Pharmaceutical Meds
- High Stress Levels
- Lack of Rest & Recovery

You can effectively neutralize many of these environmental downsides and also quiet your "bad' genes with the correct eating and lifestyle habit alterations. We'll explore exactly what these interventions are within the following chapters. However for now it's beneficial to take a look at some of the major complications chronic inflammation can cause.

Conditions

Crohn's Disease

This is more commonly known as colitis or irritable bowel syndrome (IBS). It's essentially a set of problems which arise in the digestive tracts of those who experience it. More accurately, its an irritation of the large intestine and a disorder which can cause bloating, stomach pain, abdominal cramps and even diarrhea and constipation.

In extreme cases it may develop into Ulcerative Colitis, wherein sores and ulcers form on the bowel walls. It's claimed that around 1-2 million American's are living with some degree of Crohn's disease today. This condition currently has no permanent cure, just management through proper dietary considerations like the ones described in this book and others.

Autoimmune Diseases

I have touched upon the notion of an over exaggerated inflammatory and immune response already. It's this exact situation which causes the following conditions I.e. when the immune system mistakenly begins to attack normal and healthy cells of the body. Lupus is a very common form of this type of autoimmune disorder.

Celiac disease is another one, this time causing damage to the small intestine due to an inability to process gluten properly. Psoriasis is a long lasting inflammation of the skin which causes itchy red patches all over the body. And finally Hashimoto's Disease, an autoimmune dysfunction which attacks the cells of the thyroid, leading to swelling and general gland down regulation.

Asthma

This one isn't commonly known to be an inflammation derived disease. However, it's actually caused by a set of cells known as eosinophils and neutrophils, which are inflammatory in nature and act in infiltrating the smaller airways of the lungs. This causes these narrow pathways to constrict further, reducing or even preventing airflow completely. This causes a typical asthma attack we all know so well.

Arthritis

Rheumatoid Arthritis is a condition most commonly attributed to the elderly, but can also occur in younger folks in their 20's and 30's if they develop sufficient amounts of this type of inflammation within the joints. It occurs when the synovium, a thin, specialized membrane which secretes synovial fluids into the joints to keep them lubricated, becomes overly inflamed.

Osteoarthritis is actually the form of arthritis which is due to wear and tear or joint overuse. It's caused primarily as a result of repetitive strain style injuries when a person is constantly putting a joint through the same range of motion in a stressful manner. Think in a sporting sense like tennis elbow for instance. Inflammation is sparked in order to heal the damage initially, but often persists far too long causing server pain and discomfort.

Diabetes

I have written in much greater detail with regards to diabetes and it's implications within other books such as "Insulin Resistance: A Nutritionists Guide". However, it is still very relevant for a discussion on inflammation, due to the nature of how the condition can be caused.

Essentially, a situation may arise where chronic inflammation can cause an attack on the beta cells of the pancreas. If this continues for any considerable length of time, these cells become damaged to the extent of being unable to produce insulin at all. This will result in full scale insulin dependant type 1 diabetes in extreme cases.

Heart Disease

In my experience this is the least considered form of inflammation causing conditions. Heart problems in truth are down to a number of considerations regarding the entire cardiovascular system as a whole. Although chronic inflammation is once again a culprit here, especially if it becomes localized within the coronary arteries, which encase the heart. This will exacerbate, if not be fully responsible for atherosclerosis and heart disease at some point down the line.

All of these conditions within this section, are essentially caused by the same ailment. They are due to an inappropriate and prolonged inflammation response, just realized in different locations within the body. That's the bad news. The good news is that they can all be alleviated or even cured with the same intervention measures, in a one cure fixes all type fashion.

The second part of this book will show you exactly how this is done. What dietary and lifestyle adaptations to make in order to tame any chronic inflammation you maybe experiencing. Although before doing so, we need to take a look at one more factor with regards to adequately diagnosing this condition, along with ensuring that you are under the correct medical care when attempting to fix it.

CHAPTER 3: HOW TO SEEK THE CORRECT MEDICAL HELP (IF NEEDED)

The idea for this book, and my diet and detox series in general, is to provide the dietary and lifestyle changes necessary to avoid many of the illnesses and aliments I've described in the previous chapter and others. I have seen this stuff work in countless clients, friends and family alike.

That being said, chronic inflammation is not something to be taken lightly. Although I stand by the health and wellness advice I provide, you should still be consulting your local GP and be under the guidance of these health care professionals, if you do indeed believe you are suffering from this condition.

Hence why I am including this chapter. If you are experiencing a number of the previously described symptoms, than it's a good idea to go and get checked out. Confirming your condition one way or the other is the first step on the road to recovery. It allows you to lay out a plan with regards to healing yourself.

In order to help your doctor with regards to an accurate diagnosis, it's highly beneficial to keep a log of your lifestyle for at least a couple of weeks leading up to your assessment. Keep a food diary of exactly what you have been consuming on a daily basis. Also note the exact symptoms you have been experiencing, as well as the times of day they occur.

They will then have a better idea of exactly what battery of tests to run, and what to be looking out for in a blood panel. The two main markers of general inflammation being C-Reactive Protein, which is produced by the liver and signals the onset of a range of autoimmune diseases. And Cortisol, a hormone released by the adrenal gland in response to stressful conditions within the body. It's highly anti-inflammatory and deployed to diffuse the fires being lit inside of yourself.

Who should you go and see?

There are a number of options with regards to the various practitioners available to you. This can be a little overwhelming, so I usually suggest to simply go and visit your local GP first and foremost, to get an initial read on your condition. He or she will then be able to pass you onto the correct specialist if they see fit.

These practitioners will range from specific medical doctors to naturopathic consultants such as an acupuncturist, yoga instructor or meditation coach (more on this in the following chapter). You may also see a dietary consultant or nutritionist (although hopefully this is where I can help).

But for now, lets stick with the traditional medical specialists.

Whist there isn't a specific branch of medicine which deals with inflammation exclusively, there are more standard measures these doctors will take. It actually depends on where your inflammatory disorder is manifesting, with regards to exactly who you are likely to see.

A gastroenterologist will more than likely deal with inflammation within the digestive tracts such as Crohn's and IBS. A dermatoigist will deal with cases involving the skin including Psoriasis for instance. You may even see a cardiologist if you have more serious inflammation around the coronary arteries or vasculature in general.

However, in terms of the medications these professionals prescribe, it's usually along very similar lines. They will typically advise one of the three following avenues to take with regards to the general treatment of inflammation:

1. **Non-Steroidal Anti-Inflammatory Drugs (NSAID's)**

This family of compounds are designed to both help reduce inflammation in addition to acting as pain killers in some cases. They will block certain enzymes within the system and halt the production of any inflammatory chemicals, preventing symptoms from getting any worse. You will likely know many of these drugs as the generic over the counter versions are household names I.e. Aspirin and Ibuprofen.

2. Corticosteroids

As the name suggests, this set of substances are steroid based and come in oral or injectable forms. They are naturally produced compounds within the adrenal cortex such as hydrocortisone and cortisone. Although doctors can now prescribe their synthetic analogues, which have been developed via copying their molecular structures. They are used to treat widespread chronic inflammation by deactivating genes responsible for the inflammatory response in the first place.

3. Acetaminophen

Better known as paracetamol by most, or via it's generic name Tylenol (in the US) and Panadol (in the rest of the world). This compound is primarily used to treat localized pain such as headaches or the general effects of a fever or flu. It's used as a means to reduce pain, but not prevent inflammation processes in anyway.

Like any pharmaceutical meds, just ensure you are taking the correct amount and not for too long, as they will start to cause stomach problems if abused. Always remember that these are typically short term measures. They are momentary solutions which calm the fires of chronic inflammation and mask symptoms for the most part.

This is why they are not long term solutions in the slightest. I'm not saying you shouldn't make use of these substances if you are indeed suffering in pain. Not at all. You just have to view them for what they are, simply as a means to an end. A tool to help you in the beginning while you fix the route causes of your condition.

This is where the naturopathic practitioners come in. To encourage the lifestyle measures and changes you'll have to make in order to get your health back on track. If you get this right you will fix a host of physiological and psychological problems in the process. Remember everything blends into one when it comes to overall well-being.

Healing the system as a whole is ultimately how you achieve full fitness once again. Fixing your mind and soul fixes the body and vice versa. They play into positive feedback loops which snowball your progress on the path to optimal health. So make sure you read the next chapter with a clear and open mind, as the benefits of employing such progressive measures can be immense.

PART 2: PRACTICAL WAYS TO REDUCE INFLAMMATION IN THE BODY - EVERYDAY TIPS & EATING PLANS

CHAPTER 4: LIFESTYLE INTERVENTIONS TO REDUCE INFLAMMATION NATURALLY

Alongside seeking the adequate medical help and advice for your chronic inflammation, there is also many naturopathic avenues you can explore. Your doctor may even prescribe these to you themselves, depending on how open minded they are. These will include stress relief and relaxation techniques, designed to alleviate inflammation within the body, in addition to dietary and medicinal measures.

If done correctly, they should complement one another. As I always state, the body functions as a complex set of mechanisms working in synchronicity. Everything must be kept in a healthy balance to continue working optimally. The mind is a powerful component in this puzzle and is a critical tool for the efficient working of these biological systems, as well as aiding in recovery and repair when they become damaged.

So many of these practices will lend very well to next. There is also some significant overlap with regards to these techniques and many are performed in conjunction with one another. You may in fact be actively practicing one or more of these already. My advice would be to give them a try if you are not. There is simply nothing to lose from doing so. The payoff can be huge if you find the right combination which works for you.

Yoga

Like many of these techniques, yoga is a fantastic stress reduction tool. I prescribe it to virtually all of my clients due to the plethora of health and wellness benefits it brings. Better core stability, functional strength, flexibility as well as mind muscle connection.

However, regular yoga practice has also been shown to reduce inflammation in the body, alongside these more traditional exercise benefits. It does this by stimulating a higher production of leptin and adiponectin in the body, two natural compounds which are highly affective at reducing inflammation. In addition to this, it also reduces levels of pro-inflammatory substances such as cytokines, whilst easing pain in the process.

If done correctly and consistently, you should find a restorative quality yoga will bring to the body. It will help soothe the central nervous system and drain the lymph nodes aiding overall lymphatic and blood flow around the body. Make sure you practice at least a beginner level routine for a minimum of 10 minutes per day, preferably in the morning to kick start these cleansing biological processes.

General Relaxation Techniques for Stress Reduction

Alongside yoga, its a good idea to explore some more general tactics for reducing stress on a daily basis. There are many relaxation techniques available to you. It's simply about learning how to keep your emotional levels in check, and within a tolerable and healthy range. This will help all physiological systems to continue working efficiently.

It's also the most optimal state for beneficial decision making, as the rational centers of the brain aren't inhibited by elevated sympathetic nervous system activity, which can trigger a stressful "fight or flight" response if you are not careful. This will cause a noticeable change in your physiology. It will initiate a secretion of the stress and inflammation hormones, a biological consequence of this distress.

So never miss the opportunity to relax whenever necessary. Try to keep your worries to a minimum, as excessive and pointless postulation will always lead to unnecessary stress. Breathing techniques, exercise, laughter therapy, and other methods are all available within an inflammation reducing protocol. Make it a habit to stay relaxed. Your body and mind will thank you for it I can assure you.

Mindfulness Practice

If you are looking for more specific examples of what relaxation techniques to try, then mindfulness training is a good place to start. Mindfulness is defined as the awareness of the present, both in terms of moment and circumstance. Deriving its roots from Buddhism, it actually seems like an oxymoronic statement at first. "Mindfulness" sounds like the mind is "full" of thoughts, when the exact opposite is the case. It simply means being very careful with your thoughts, and to hold none whatsoever for most of the day.

This clarity of mind concept has gained all sorts of contemporary applications in today's world, both in the fields of psychology and new age self-help circles. It has been proven to be extremely effective in both managing highly stressful situations, as well as the cascade of emotions and negative hormonal consequences such circumstances can promote.

But how can you practice this for yourself? Firstly, you have to pay attention to everything that's occurring around you, all of the sights, sounds and distractions. Then it's about focusing on just one element of your environment, like your breath, in order to enter a somewhat peaceful mediation state. But most importantly, to ensure that you keep all of your focus on the present moment.

Mindfulness is not an easy thing to master, but once you do so, its a powerful tool. If you find it too tricky at first, you can seek the help of an expert to guide you in your mindfulness training. There are many excellent books on this topic which delve into it's practices and benefits in much greater detail than I can here.

So my advice is to do your research and start down the road on your mindful journey. It will help with better mental clarity and reduce worries and anxiety throughout the day. It's the starting point of my next stress reduction technique.

Meditation

There are many types of meditation practices available to you such as ascension, transcendental and guerilla mediation, just to name a few. Science is continually revealing the positive benefits of performing regular mediation sessions, such as reducing levels of depression and post traumatic stress disorders, as well as an increase in overall brain function and improved creativity.

Studies are now confirming a correlative increase in gray matter within the outer cortexes of the brain, a neuroplasticity adaptation resulting from regular mediation. It has also been shown to help dampen or even switch off inflammation causing genes in the first place.

There is simply no reason not to incorporate this into your day. Try allocating a time when you are most likely to be uninterrupted. Again, first thing in the morning perhaps and/or late at night. However, you can always find a quiet spot anywhere during the day to practice meditation, like an empty room or the bathroom if you want an added boost.

Start by initially focusing on your breath once more. Breathing techniques can be performed as a calming practice in and of themselves, or as part of a mediation session. Slow and steady breaths not only calms the mind, but have significant physiological benefits such as flooding the body with oxygen, whilst simultaneously removing toxic carbon dioxide.

Simply meditate and calm yourself often. Your focus should be on peace and positivity when doing so. Positive attitude affirmations work best for me, although a complete clearing of the mind in a mindfulness type session works best for others. Regardless, it will help to re-set your psyche, and recharge the central nervous system when done correctly.

Exercise

I go into greater detail with regards to exercise protocols within "Intermittent Fasting" & "Sugar Detox: A Nutritionists Guide". But suffice to say that incorporating at least some form of physical activity into your daily or weekly routine is essential. Certainly if improved health and wellness levels is the goal.

With regards to inflammation specifically, researchers are now finding that along with reducing other chronic diseases such as arthritis, obesity and diabetes. Regular exercise is also effective in producing an anti-inflammatory cellular response within the body. A precursor to many of the conditions in the first place.

It also does not require a significant amount of work to produce these beneficial effects, just 20 minutes of moderate exercise such as jogging, cycling or swimming has been shown to be effective in eliciting these adaptations.

If you are not used to doing these types of workouts, than simply start slowly. Build 2-3 of these sessions into your week to begin with. Once conditioned to the workload, up the frequency to 20-30 minutes everyday if you can. In truth, any amount of physical activity above and beyond what you are currently doing will be beneficial.

Of course, if you are suffering from any severe illness or condition already, then get the clearance from your personal physician or local GP before doing so.

Rest & Recovery

The final consideration when it comes to overall health, is adequate rest and recovery. This is overlooked by so many people in today's society. It's understandable with the hectic lives we lead. I often reduce peoples workloads in the gym if I think they aren't getting adequate rest for any reason.

Downtime is when the body heals itself. It's when it repairs from physical activity, when the muscles grow after heavy workouts.

Impeding this recovery prevents these improvements and adaptations from taking place. It keeps you in the same spot, perpetually unable to progress not matter how hard you are training.

I write in greater detail with regards to metabolic damage with my book on insulin resistance, but it's safe to say that getting sufficient rest is paramount for full and proper recovery! There is such a thing as over training, and while the average person will unlikely ever exceed the scientific definition of this condition, we all work ourselves too hard and for too long from time to time.

Sleep is a big part of this. Ensure you are getting at least 8 hours a night. Some of you may require slightly less, some a fraction more. But this has been proven to be the optimal range I.e. 7-9 hours, for complete recovery in terms of tissue repair, memory restoration, central nervous system re-set and appetite control.

So ensure you are taking these lifestyle considerations on board. Increase the amount of relaxation and meditation exercises you are performing each day. This is the start on the road to clearing the toxins and pathogens from the body.

However, getting a good grasp on your diet will ultimately be the key to controlling inflammation within the system. This is why the reminder of this book will focus primarily on these nutritional elements, to most optimally eradicate inflammation from the body once and for all.

CHAPTER 5: REMEMBER FOOD IS THY MEDICINE

"It's the food… Its' always been the food!"

(Dr Michael Klaper)

Before we get onto the specifics with regards to what to be consuming on an anti-inflammatory style diet plan, it's beneficial to explore some of the higher level principles when it comes to healthy eating. This is a combination of some of my personal feelings and the scientific discoveries which have been made over the years.

I have mentioned this within other books. But for quite some time now, governments and the research community have been strongly recommending people to cut back on the overall saturated fat and cholesterol intake within their diets. This is for good reason. Contrary to what the egg and meat industry funded studies show, there is a high causal link between consumption of these types of foods, and the degenerative diseases we face today. Heart attacks, strokes etc. The clinical data is very clear on this.

Unhealthy food causes inflammation within the system, plain and simple. It takes the body a lot of effort to deal with these substances, not only in terms of digestion, but also to heal the damage they cause in the process. Some of these food sources such as red meat, are even being re-categorized as type 1 carcinogens, due to the potential cancer risks they pose.

Of course there will be slight variations in a persons dietary habits with regards to exactly what they are trying to achieve I.e. weight loss, sugar detoxing, insulin resistance, inflammation reduction etc. However, there are certainly some overarching principles to abide by. Healthy eating has some fundamental do's and don'ts which apply to all of the above dietary protocols.

My advice is always to switch to clean and unprocessed sources of produce. More on this in the following two chapters. But for now, lets just say that you should be focusing on the fresh fruit and vegetable aisles much more than you probably have been. Cancer research foundations all around the world are continually increasing the amounts of vitamins and oxidants required from these foods, just to stave off the disease. Typically 10-13 serving a day now!

A wide ranging and colorful collection of fruits and vegetables provides all of the micro nutrients we require to remain healthy. They also provide the fiber and roughage to aid digestion in a big way, and most importantly, are highly anti-inflammatory. The typical "Standard American" diet simply does not contain enough of these disease fighting food substances. This is the first thing to get right.

Then it's about selecting the correct sources of healthy fats, proteins and carbohydrates in order to get your macro nutrient profile right. Again, this will differ slightly with regards to the health and fitness goals you are trying to achieve. Obtaining healthy sources of fats from omega-3 rich avocados and wild caught fish is a must though. Consuming lean sources of protein from nuts and poultry is paramount. Eating high grade low GI carbs from whole grains such as brown rice, quinoa and simple oats is key.

All of these food sources provide adequate energy and nutrition in and of themselves. They all serve a purpose with regards to energy provision or nutrient supply. Avoiding "empty calorie" foods on the other hand is a must, as they do the opposite. Processed sugary sweets and snacks provide no nutritional value, spike blood sugar levels followed by the inevitably crash. They keep you on the sugar rush roller coaster!

Don't worry here if you are feeling a little lost on what you should be doing. I have your back on this. The following chapter will delve into greater detail with regards to the specific food items to place in your grocery basket each week, and which ones to avoid like the plague. So grab a pen a paper and let's get this sorted.

CHAPTER 6: A WORD ON PESTICIDES - CLEAN FIFTEEN VS DIRTY DOZEN

"Processed foods cause inflammation, a source of most illnesses as well as stress"

(Kris Carr)

As we have discussed within the previous chapter regarding overall healthy eating, consuming high amounts of fresh produce in the form of fruits and vegetables is the key to health and well-being in the long run. In reality, eating these foods from any sources is beneficial, due to the free radical eliminating and cancer fighting properties they provide, in the form of vitamins and antioxidants.

However, we do need to be somewhat cautious when attempting to optimize this anti-inflammatory response. This is due to one consideration, which are the pesticides these foods may contain. Unfortunately many of the fruits and vegetables we buy today are coated in pesticide residue, in order to protect them from being eaten by insects whilst they're grown.

These chemicals aren't good. They increase a farmers produce yield, but at what cost to the consumer? It's only starting to become clear what the specific health implications of consuming too much of this stuff can do to the body. Pesticides have been shown to irritate the human digestive system and cause inflammation within the cells and tissues.

Of course going fully organic is your best option here, although I know this can be the more expensive option in most cases. Again, you really have to decide what is important in life. If you can manage to cut back in other areas in order to afford those higher priced apples and bell peppers, then do it.

If you simply want to reduce your exposure to these chemicals, then it's a good idea to stick to the "clean fifteen" list of foods, whilst avoiding the "dirty dozen". These foods do change slightly from year to year as farming practices improve or deteriorate in the various regions of the world where they are produced. But it's a good guide to abide by nonetheless.

Simply put, the foods on the clean fifteen list are the ones which take the least amount of chemicals and pesticides to produce. Whilst the dirty dozen typically require higher amounts in order to get them into the supermarket and onto your plate.

This data is actually comprised by a nonprofit watchdog organization named the Environmental Working Group (EWG). Each year they compile data from the US Department of Agriculture (USDA), and the Food and Drug Administration (FDA) regarding these pesticide figures.

So firstly, lets start with the good stuff. What you should be putting into your grocery basket each week:

Clean Fifteen (2017 list)

- Avocados
- Asparagus
- Cabbage
- Cantaloupe
- Cauliflower
- Eggplant
- Grapefruit
- Honeydew
- Kiwifruit
- Mangoes
- Onions
- Papayas
- Pineapples
- Sweet Corn
- Sweet Peas

Dirty Dozen (2017 list)

Now lets take a look at what you should ideally be avoiding. If you absolutely have to buy these foods for your favorite meals, then try to stick to the organic options of the following if you can:

- Apples
- Celery
- Cherries
- Grapes
- Nectarines
- Peaches
- Pears
- Potatoes
- Spinach
- Strawberries
- Sweet bell peppers
- Tomatoes

Of course these lists are just guidelines and they do change from time to time, so ensure you keep an updated list on the refrigerator door each year. Try to stick to them as much as possible in order to reduce this inflammation producing pesticide response. Also make sure you are washing everything thoroughly with water before cooking and consuming to further reduce any chemical residue.

Local farmers markets are your best bet if you happen to have some high quality producers in and around your area. This will be heavily seasonally dependant, which is a good thing, as at least you know you are getting the most nutritional bang for your buck.

The fruits and vegetables haven't had to travel far and wide to get to you. Reducing the need for pesticides during production, as well as chemicals to preserve the produce during transportation.

Like organic options, these farms will be a little more expensive compared to buying them within your local supermarket for instance. But again, just do what you can. Don't over think this stuff to begin with. Just make the best possible choices as and when you can.

CHAPTER 7: REMOVING GLUTEN & DIARY - A GAME CHANGER

"One of the easiest and most effective ways of reducing inflammation, is by fueling your body with food that supports you"

(Eva Selhub MD)

So having looked at the first layer of defence when it comes to eliminating inflammation in the body I.e. reducing the chemical and pesticide load contained within the foods we are eating. It's now time to look at a second set of factors with regards to whats on our plate. To investigate two of the worst culprits for aggravating inflammatory factors.

These are gluten and dairy. You have no doubt heard of the downsides of these food sources from countless people in the past. They are usually just regurgitating what they have heard online somewhere or from a friend who managed to cut them out of their diet successfully. I'm not against anecdotal evidence entirely, especially if it comes from trusted sources like close friends and family for instance.

But it's wise to take a look at some of the hard and fast facts when it comes to these two food substances. So you can make the most well informed decision on whether to remove them completely from your own diet or not. This is ultimately up to you. My advice to anyone suffering from even mild inflammation causing conditions, is to go cold turkey on these to begin with, to see how your body responds.

Gluten

Gluten is a substance which can be found in many of the foods we consume on a daily basis. It's actually a protein contained within most wheat products and commonly found in barley, rye, wheat germ, kamut, bulgur, farro, semolina and so on. Gliadin is actually the problem protein more specifically, as it sets off an immune response in the small intestine destroying microvilli and impeding nutrient absorption.

Those with Celiac disease are the worst effected by this food substrate. Gluten aggravates their digestive tracts and causes many forms of inflammatory conditions. Even those without the disorder can still suffer the ill consequences on consuming too much gluten containing foods. Along with the digestive issues, you may also experience sinus problems, joint pain, headaches, blood sugar imbalances, hormonal anomalies and skin conditions.

We will get into greater detail with regards to specific food sources to consume and avoid in the following chapter, but for now, lets just say that skipping gluten containing meals is a good idea. The easiest way to do this is by removing any grains from your diet which aren't gluten free. Avoid the sources I've already listed here for a start.

This will include many of your favorite foods most probably. Breads, cakes, bagels, cereals, cookies, pizza's, pasta and the like. Essentially anything which contains common wheat flour as its main ingredient. Also look for more "hidden" sources of gluten contained within barley, malts, beers, brewers yeast, brown flour, dextrin, syrups and modified starches.

This will take a bit of label scrutiny to begin with. It will require some fact checking with regards to the typical foods you are buying and consuming. But it will be time worth spent, as the reduction in inflammation you will see as a result of eradicating these substances from your diet can be immense.

You have two options in reality. The first is to simply remove all of these food groups from your daily meals. This is the safest option, although I know this can seem very exclusive and an extreme thing to do at first. The second option is to stick to "gluten free" products, which are now plentiful within the stores and supermarkets you'll frequent.

Again, simply check the labels for "gluten free", "without gluten" or "no gluten" clearly stated on them. The FDA and food allergens associations are very hot on ensuring these standards are met if a company is stating any of these terms on their packaging. They will typically contain the "Certified Gluten Free" symbol somewhere on the packaging also, as an extra fail safe measure when selecting these foods.

Dairy

This is the other "bad guy" when it comes to pinpointing the cause of inflammation inducing dietary components, especially with regards to digestive tract issues once again. I have written in greater detail within "Sugar Detox: A Nutritionists Guide" relating the ill effects of consuming dairy on the human body.

But to summarize again for you here. Most folks don't produce nearly enough of the enzyme lactase to properly breakdown the lactose in the system, a disaccharide which is formed via a combination of glucose and galactose. Lactose is widely known as the "milk sugar".

Whilst this is officially termed as lactose intolerance, for those medically diagnosed with the condition. Large portions of the population are also very much ill-equipped to deal with lactose to varying degrees. Meaning they will experience the downsides of this condition to some level if they are eating these types of foods consistently. Digestive problems, bloating and possible diarrhea can all follow.

Typical food sources which contain lactose include milk, infant formula, ice cream, yogurt, and custard. Essentially any dairy product. These should be avoided if you are seriously attempting to eradicate inflammation in the system. They are mucus producing foods which coat the lining of the intestines preventing nutrient uptake.

I know this will be the biggest hurdle for most people when it comes to switching to an anti-inflammatory diet, or any healthy eating plan for that matter. The thought of giving up dairy is often too much to bear, especially in the minds of those cheese lovers.

But if you think about it, apart from the taste, what is to like? Traditional cows milk is the mammary secretion of a bovine animal, not meant for us in the first place. It's designed to grow a baby calf from around 80 lbs at birth, to more than 240 lbs in just three months I.e. tripling its weight.

It's loaded with fats, as well as growth hormones and synthetic antibiotics artificially fed to the female cows whilst producing this stuff. All of which further increases the inflammation response within us when we drink it.

For me, this was an easy one to give up. I never enjoyed the taste of raw milk or cheese to begin with. I recall spending entire playtime's in primary school agonizingly sipping on cartoons of warm milk our teachers would force us drink before being allowed to run around outside. They of course didn't know any better, and presumed it was good for our bone development and overall health.

I'll spare you the dietary calcium studies which point to the opposite I.e. calcium derived from dairy may actually bleed it from the system, causing an overall increase in bone fracture incidents. You are much better off getting this essential mineral from dark leafy greens. I certainly would have preferred a kale or spinach smoothie growing up!

Nowadays it's obviously much easier to manage these things more appropriately in my diet. I'm not perfect by any means, and still do consume the odd cheese topped pizza or ice cream from time to time. But its extremely rare and I always feel tired, bloated and regretful after doing so.

Much the same as gluten, my advice would be to cut out dairy completely to begin with if you are suffering severe symptoms of dietary induced inflammation, as its almost certainly a major cause of this distress. At least cut down the amounts you are consuming considerably. You should notice the difference in the way you feel immediately when you do so.

CHAPTER 8: OTHER FOOD GROUPS TO INCLUDE & AVOID

"Include in your diet plenty of vegetables, and if possible, at least a glass of raw vegetable juice per day"

(Dr. Royal Lee)

Obtaining some outline meal guides is essential for getting your anti-inflammatory diet off to a good start. But before we get into the recipes though, its wise to assess some more individual food sources in order to know exactly what we should be including in them. It's beneficial to eradicate some more culprits causing this inflammation, but also to add in the components which help us bring it down.

Some Substances to Avoid

We have already noted that gluten and dairy are the two main food components to remove from our diet first and foremost. However, the following list should also be withdrawn or certainly consumed with care, when trying to eliminate inflammatory responses in the body:

Caffeine

High caffeine levels in the system can cause a number of issues when it comes to digestion. A strong coffee will stimulate the stomach to eject its contents faster than it ordinarily would, forcing semi-digested food into the small intestine. This can have an aggravating effect on the digestive tract in general.

Excess caffeine can also spike blood sugar levels, increase heart rate and blood pressure, as well as suppressing appetite. It will also put stress on the central nervous system impeding the production and efficiency of Cortisol, the body's primary anti-inflammatory hormone.

Alcohol

This is quite an obvious one to quash in truth. A glass of red wine with your meals every now and then won't do too much harm, even provide some additional antioxidants. But consuming copious amounts of alcohol in general, will not only provide excess sugar loads to spike blood glucose once more, it will also increase C-Reactive Protein levels in the system.

Excessive amounts of alcoholic beverages will damage gut flora also, leading to poor digestive functioning known as a "leaking gut". Food will find it difficult to break through the intestinal walls, whilst simultaneously inducing an immune system response. This can further stimulate inflammation and allergies within the body.

Eggs

Eggs have been touted as one of the ultimate health foods for many years now. But are they really that good for us? Yes they do contain a lot of nutritional bang for their buck in terms of calorie load. But similar to the considerations regarding animal products in general, they carry a high saturated fat content (if you are consuming the yolks). They also contain around 6 grams of pure protein per egg white.

However, they are very high in inflammatory omega-6 fatty acids, in addition to containing far fewer disease fighting and anti-cancer vitamins and antioxidants, compared with their plant counterparts. There is also a chance of contracting salmonella poisoning if you are not cooking or storing your eggs properly.

I know this one all to well as I experienced it on a trip to South East Asia a few years back, whilst on holiday in Thailand. I started to feel intense stomach pains after consuming an omelet one morning, and it took me 3 days to get over the excruciating agony in a Bangkok hospital…

Known Allergens

Finally, it's a good idea to steer clear of the top allergen food sources if you can. Or again, at least cut back on them as much as possible. These substances will effect everyone to varying degrees, but have been shown to elicit immune aggravating properties across the board. We have covered three of these already in wheat, dairy and eggs. But also included in this list would be peanuts and shellfish I.e. crab, shrimps and lobster.

Top Inflammation Fighting Foods & Herbs

So having highlighted some of the food sources to eradicate, lets now take a look at some of the best options to include in your dishes. These food substances which will help calm the fires on chronic inflammation within the body:

Dark Leafy Greens

Kale, spinach, arugula and bok choy all contain very high quantities of vitamin E, which has an anti-inflammatory effect on the body. It diffuses inflammation causing molecules such as cytokines and free radicals. These food sources help repair cell and tissue damage caused by these molecules, as well as having a distinct anti-aging effect on the skin via collagen and elastin restoration within the dermis layer.

Dark leafy greens also contain high levels of calcium and vitamin K, both key components when it comes to bone health. So swap out that class of milk for a green smoothie and your chances of breaking any bones will go down with it.

Wild Caught Salmon

In reality you can include any forms of oily fish such as mackerel, pilchards and sardines into your dishes if you choose. All of these fish species contain high levels of anti-inflammatory omega-3 fatty acids. Salmon is my favorite though, not only due to the taste, but as it also contains potent disease fighting levels of vitamin b12, vitamin D and selenium.

Just make sure to avoid the larger fish species such as tuna, halibut and monkfish as they contain higher than recommended levels of mercury.

Whole Grains

I have written at length with regards to the extensive qualities of consuming lots of whole grains within your diet. Brown rice, quinoa, millet and simple oats are low GI carbs which contain high levels of fiber, slowing down digestion and reducing high blood sugar spikes. They release energy more slowly throughout the day reducing additional food cravings, especially for sugary and sweet snacks.

Whole grains are also extremely anti-inflammatory, as they have been shown to reduce C-Reactive Protein levels in the body. High grade whole grains will also reduce overall risk of strokes, diabetes and heart disease. Just make sure the grains you are consuming come from gluten free sources.

Blueberries & Cranberries

Berries in general are some of the best superfoods available to us. They contain extremely high levels of cancer fighting and anti-inflammatory phytonutrients such as flavonoids and anthocyanin pigments.

You can also include tart cherries into this group. In addition to being extremely sweet and tasty, cherries also contain high anti-inflammatory compounds. I never go a day without at least one large fruit smoothie (typically to start the day) containing a mixed cup full of these awesome little berries and cherries.

Nuts & Seeds

Nuts and seeds are also very high fiber foods, once again aiding with overall digestion. They also contain large amounts of vitamin E, and omega-3 fatty acids contributing to the conversion of healthy DHA and EPA within the body.

My favorite nut sources are walnuts and almonds as they also contain manganese. My top sources of seeds being chia, hemp and flaxseeds. Make sure you also add a teaspoon of each of these within your smoothies to garner the additional benefits they provide.

Garlic

Depending on your preference for its taste, garlic is a great addition to many meals due to it's anti-inflammatory and immune boosting properties. It has also been shown to protect against many forms digestive tract cancers. If you do not like to consume garlic in your foods, you can always supplement with tasteless capsules if needed.

Broccoli

A stable vegetable for almost any occasion, broccoli is highly anti-inflammatory. It contains beneficial phytonutrients such sulforaphane and kaempferol which reduce inflammation and oxidative stress within the body. Broccoli also contains significant levels of vitamin C, as well as potassium and magnesium, all compounds which further promote overall health and well-being.

Celery

Celery is commonly thought to be devoid of much nutritional content, although this is a myth. Like broccoli, it contains many phytonutrients and cancer fighting antioxidants which diffuse inflammation and oxidative stress. These include vitamin C once more, beta-carotene and manganese. One of my favourite snacks is to dip a stick of celery into an unsweetened tub of natural peanut butter! Just be careful to wash your celery thoroughly beforehand, as it's regularly on the dirty dozen list.

Turmeric

Unless you have been living under a rock for the past few years, you will certainly have heard about the abundant health properties of this amazing yellow herb. Turmeric via its active compound curcumin, heavily reduces inflammation and swelling in the body, alleviating symptoms of osteoarthritis and arthritis within the joints.

It also has anti-cancer properties as well as helping to reduce digestive problems in the stomach and intestines. There is literally no reason not to include this earthy powder in your dishes. I even include a teaspoon in my shakes as well. My knee pain always disappears when I do.

Ginger

Along with turmeric, ginger is thought to be the other potent anti-inflammatory powerhouse available in natural food form. In combination, these two substances have been found to be as effective (if not more so) than some of the non-steroidal drugs we have already mentioned.

They have immense healing properties which help soothe the root cause of the inflammation within the body, and not simply mask symptoms. I now add ginger to all of my herbal teas, as well as green apple, carrot and ginger juices. It helps them taste great and gives me that added anti-inflammatory effect.

This list is certainly not exhaustive, but just a guide to show you some of the best immune supporting and anti-inflammatory foods which have been proven to be effective. In truth, consuming a wide variety of organic and fresh produce will stand you in good stead. The aforementioned list are just some of the food sources to try and include when and where you can.

ANTI-INFLAMMATORY DIET

Some other noteworthy mentions would be avocados, onions, red cabbage, pineapples, papaya's, olive and coconut oil. All of these foods contain additional elements of the vitamins, minerals and antioxidants necessary to help calm any inflammation in the body. The following chapter will give you an idea on how to put some of these combinations together to complete the anti-inflammatory dietary play book.

CHAPTER 9: MEAL PLANS - VEGAN, PALEO & MEDITERRANEAN OPTIONS

"Flavour fresh, real food. You can be assured that you are offering your body anti-inflammatory nutrition"

(Deepak Chopra)

It's now time to take a look at some specific anti-inflammatory meal plans, in order to give you an idea of what to prepare on a daily basis. As always, this will just be a guiding framework. Something you can base your own dishes around with regards to your personal tastes and preferences. This is the key to making it work for you.

There are a number of options here depending on your inclinations. This is the good thing about an anti-inflammatory style diet, or any healthy eating plan for that matter. If you know the basics, you can plan the individual components of your dishes in line with your preferences I.e. Paleo, Mediterranean or Vegan style options.

The following will give you an idea of what you should be including in each of these food categories. As always, these are simply suggestions. You may want to copy my dishes to begin with, but slowly expanding on them over time is the best way to ensure adherence to the diet in order to stay the course.

Vegan Options

Breakfast:

Mixed Greens & Berry Smoothie

A handful of kale & spinach,
One chopped banana,
1/2 cup of simple oats,
Some shredded coconut,
1 cup of mixed frozen berries,
1 scoop of chocolate vegan protein power,
1 teaspoon of chia, hemp & flaxseeds,
Mixed with water.

Lunch:

Spinach & Shiitake Mushroom Pasta

2 large shiitake mushrooms
1/2 cup of diced baby spinach,
1 teaspoon of canola oil,
Crushed garlic, Dijon mustard or white wine vinegar,
On top of some whole grain spaghetti pasta.

ANTI-INFLAMMATORY DIET

Dinner:

Sweet Potato Chilli

1 medium sized boiled sweet potato,
1 cup of mixed cannellini & kidney beans,
1 chopped red pepper,
1 diced red onion,
Oregano, cumin & paprika,
On top of 1/2 cup of gluten free white rice.

Snack:

Celery sticks dipped in raw peanut butter.

Paleo Options

Breakfast:

Pomegranate & Berry Smoothie

1 cup of unsweetened almond milk,
1 frozen banana,
1/2 cup of pomegranate seeds,

1 cup of mixed frozen berries,
2 medjool dates,
1 teaspoon a chia, hemp & flaxseeds.

Lunch:

Coconut Milk Chicken

Slow cooked chicken thighs/drumsticks,
With garlic, cumin, coriander and turmeric,
Mixed with coconut milk and lime zest,
Served with a mixture of green vegetables.

Dinner:

Orange & Rosemary Salmon

Take one large salmon fillet,
Sear in a pan with orange juice, lime zest, garlic & fresh rosemary,
Add 1 medium sized sweet potato (mashed),
With bunch of steamed asparagus.

Snack:

Handful of 100% dark chocolate coated almonds.

As you can probably tell, this isn't a typical Paleo meal guide. It's adapted towards the "healthier" anti-inflammatory end of the spectrum. There is no red meat options due to their high saturated fat contents, and also no butter for the same reason. In addition to this, I have also included a vegetable component to each dish to increase the micro-nutrient content of the meal.

Mediterranean Options

Breakfast:

Zucchini & Tomato Omelette

3 eggs whites (1 yolk),
1 thinly sliced zucchini,
1/2 cup of chopped cherry tomatoes,
Some crushed walnuts,
1 teaspoon of extra virgin olive oil,
Broiled with some salt & pepper seasoning.

Lunch:

Mediterranean Mackerel Salad

Chopped Mackerel,
1 cup of mixed beans (chick peas, black beans & kidney beans)
1 diced green bell pepper,
1 finely chopped red onion,
Topped with fresh parsley and capers,
A drizzle of extra virgin olive oil,
With 1 slice of gluten free whole grain bread.

Dinner:

Grilled Chicken & Quinoa Salad

1 grilled chicken breast,
1 large sliced red chilli,
2 crushed garlic cloves,
A handful of chopped cherry tomatoes,
1 diced red onion,
Topped with fresh mint leaves and lime zest,
A drizzle of extra virgin olive oil,
On top of 1 cup of a boiled quinoa base.

Snack:

Cucumber and carrot slices with homemade hummus dip,
With two whole grain seeded crackers.

So those are some options and outline guidelines for each avenue of food category. You can either choose to stick to one method of eating, or incorporate a mixture of these dishes into your own meal plans depending on your ethics and taste preferences.

This of course isn't meant to be an all encompassing list of meal plans to stick to. I'm not trying to produce cookbooks in this series, but rather provide the overarching principles to why and how you should be changing your eating and lifestyle habits. To adjust your diet to achieve the health goals specific to you, and layout some simple recipes to get you heading in the right direction.

There are many online sources to look up endless meal plans and information on how to prepare them if you need to. You can honestly get lost for days if you are not careful though. So my advice is to always keep it simple to begin with. Master a handful of dishes which contain your favourite foods and become great at cooking them. Then you can expand from there and add some more variety in the future.

SUMMARY

"The problem is that we are not eating food anymore. We are eating food like products"

(Dr. Alejandro Junger)

I really like this quote as it sums up the problem with just about every degenerative disease and condition we face in society today. Whether that's obesity, insulin resistance or inflammation within the body. It starts with what we are putting into our mouths. It's the fuel we are using to run our biological machinery, which determines the overall efficiency of how we function. But also the body's ability to stave off these diseases.

It doesn't matter if you own a Ferrari. If you fill the tank up with muddy water, you aren't going to get anywhere fast. In fact, you are likely to cause much more harm than good, and sooner rather than later. With regards to the human body, this damage is almost always the result of some form of chronic inflammation to begin with.

As we have seen, a short burst of acute inflammation is beneficial. It's a natural process which helps the body rid itself of pathogens and toxins, as well as stimulate the healing and repair mechanisms. The problem comes when these responses start escalate and endure. This is when chronic inflammation and autoimmune diseases can set in.

If you notice that you are experiencing prolonged swelling, bloating, excessive soreness, pain or overheating in your body. Then it's a good idea to go and get checked out, as these are the early warning signs for an onset of inflammatory conditions. If left untreated, this can easily lead onto more serious disorders such as Crohn's disease, IBS, Hashimoto's and Lupus.

Seeking the adequate medical help at this point is paramount. There are a number of steroidal and non-steroidal options available to help with the pains and symptoms initially. But remember, GP's are trained to simply look out for general conditions. As their name suggests, they are "general practitioners" designed to screen for and diagnose basic ailments within the body. So you will more than likely be passed onto a specialist depending on what type of autoimmune disorder you are experiencing.

Regardless of the medical treatments you may undergo, I would highly recommend exploring the naturopathic and lifestyle practitioners as well. Or at least be attempting some of their techniques by yourself. The relaxation and stress reduction benefits of yoga, mindfulness and mediation sessions can't be ignored. They soothe the mind and body within the hectic world we live in.

This will also include physical exercise. Studies indicate that performing just one moderate intensity session of jogging, cycling or swimming a week, is enough to produce positive anti-inflammatory improvements in the body. Alongside the more typical benefits such as lowering blood pressure and cholesterol levels, exercise has been shown to activate immunological responses too. It increases the production of cytokines and proteins such as TNF, which regulates local systemic inflammation.

Exercise will also help boost immune function and restore proper hormonal balance, in addition to improving mental and cognitive dispositions via the production of "feel good" endorphin chemicals within the brain.

This is why I have included a chapter from "Insulin Resistance" at the end of this book, with regards to progressive workout routines. Many of the physical activity considerations are universal with regards to any health and fitness goals, especially for the average person. Yes athletes and sports people require specialized programs to develop certain traits, but the exercise tips contained within that chapter work across the board for increasing overall well-being. They certainly serve as a good starting point.

In fact, you only really need to perform the morning steady paced cardio style routines to elicit the anti-inflammatory responses you are looking for. For those with slightly loftier fitness goals, I.e. strength, power or muscle hypertrophy, then by all means start to incorporate the HIIT style sessions into your week as well.

However, if you do suspect or know that you have some chronic forms of inflammation causing conditions, then ensure you get the clearance from your doctor before performing any intense physical activity. You will likely only improve your symptoms once you get yourself moving more regularly, but better to get the all clear first.

Then its about properly recovering from this physical activity. Its about getting adequate rest and restoring the body regardless of what you are doing. All of our lives can become stressful and overbearing at one point or another. You have to make sure you give your biological and mental systems enough downtime to re-set and recharge to stave off any further inflammation within the body.

That being said, the point of this book and series in general, is to focus on the most important factor of all when it comes to diffusing inflammation, which is diet. It begins with identifying any chemically laden and high pesticide containing foods. You can make good strides by closely sticking to the clean fifteen and dirty dozen lists each year, as well as washing your food thoroughly and buying organic as much as possible.

It's then about eradicating the two biggest culprits of inflammation we know today I.e. gluten and diary. This can seem extreme to those initially trying out an anti-inflammatory style eating plan. But removing these two food sources from your diet, can be a game changer in terms of reducing or even eliminating your symptoms.

There are some other food groups to try and avoid like the known allergens. There are also some key anti-inflammatory sources to ensure you are including in your meal plans, essentially heaps of fresh fruits and vegetables! If you loosely abide by these guidelines than you should be good to go. Just play around with some of the recipes and dishes to see what best fits your own taste buds.

CONCLUSION

"It's not about perfect. It's about effort. And when you bring that effort every single day, that's where transformation happens. That's how change occurs"

(Jillian Michaels)

Eradicating inflammation within the body is a marathon, not a sprint. It requires prolonged effort and adherence to make it work. It requires consistency and persistence in putting these positive lifestyle habits into action each day. The upside to doing this can be huge. More efficient digestion, increased energy levels, better sleep, a reduction in aches and pains, as well as an optimally functioning immune system.

The dietary tips contained within this book should help you to achieve this, or at least get you on your way. To aid you in alleviating inflammation and autoimmune disorders across the board. They will help diffuse Crohn's disease, Hashimotos, Psoriasis and Lupus. They will reduce the swelling and joint pain caused by osteoarthritis and arthritis.

This is why I love healthy eating so much in general, as it's a one size fits all measure approach to healing damage and inflammation anywhere in the body. Yes you will have to alter things slightly, to meet your own set of conditions. But its the one thing which has the biggest payoff over time. Food should heal not harm, and unfortunately our societies seem to have gotten this the wrong way round in recent decades.

The good news is that you can now put this right. To get yourself heading down the correct nutritional path. Hopefully I have given you some insight and guidance on how to do this. So don't just read over this material and do nothing. That would be a waste. Try implementing some of the relaxation measures and meal plans today.

Don't worry, we all slip up every now and again. The idea is to get this right for the majority of the time. To live and eat in the correct manner for at least 90% of your week. This is how you will alleviate the worst of any inflammatory problems within the body, whilst leaving a little wiggle room to stay sane if you need it. Healthy eating is a process, and one so worth getting started with, as the stakes can be high. So enjoy this journey and I wish you every success along the way.

Simon

BONUS CHAPTER

(From "Insulin Resistance : A Nutritionists Guide")

CHAPTER 8: EXERCISE PROTOCOLS - IMPROVING INSULIN SENSITIVITY

The body likes to burn sugars for fuel, plain and simple. Performing any type of physical activity utilizes high amounts of this liver and muscle glycogen. After a heavy workout session, the body replenishes these glycogen stores with glucose from the bloodstream. It momentarily increases the body's insulin sensitivity, especially with regards to skeletal muscle uptake.

The fact that exercise reduces insulin resistance isn't in question. However, there is still some debate as to which types of training methods are best for eliciting these metabolic improvements within the body.

Avenue 1 - Slow Twitch Recruitment

I have seen studies which indicate that performing prolonged, cardiovascular type endurance exercise works best for this. Training at around 50% of VO2 Max, or 60-70% maximum heart rate.

This type of activity recruits predominantly (type 1) slow twitch, aerobic muscle fibers. You know the sort, medium intensity and even paced jogging, cycling, swimming etc. You just have to hop on one of the cardio machines in the gym, a treadmill, bike, rower or cross-trainer. Just line up your favorite playlist, put in your ear phones and you're good to go!

In my experience, these types of workouts are best suited for fasted cardio style routines in the morning, when insulin sensitivity is naturally at it's highest. People often employ this type of intermittent fasting style training when weight loss is the main goal. There are plenty of benefits to fasting if done correctly. Although I wouldn't recommend it here, as we are attempting to keep blood sugar levels as stable as possible.

But in general, lengthy cardio style activity allows the body to metabolize fat molecules much more easily, due to high oxidation ratios at these intensity levels. In essences, it takes many more oxygen molecules to oxidize one molecule of fat, compared to a molecule of glucose for instance. This allows fat to be utilized much more efficiently during these less intense but prolonged workouts.

A good way to know if you are in the right output range, is to try talking to someone whilst you are working away. If it's possible to have a conversation, but it starts to become slightly uncomfortable, that's the sweet spot. Anything more intense than this and it will become increasingly more difficult to get enough oxygen into the lungs and system for what you are trying to achieve.

Avenue 2 - Fast Twitch Recruitment

I have also seen insulin resistance intervention studies work very well when putting participants on more high intensity, anaerobic circuit/sprint and weight training style workouts. When performing these HIIT I.e. High, Intensity, Interval, Training style workouts, the body switches to using more fast twitch muscle fibers.

This forces the body to begin metabolizing glucose almost exclusively as its energy substrate, as there is now much less oxygen circulating within the system. It simply has no other choice. It will also predominantly utilize this glycogen from intra-muscular stores as it's the most readily available source during this time.

The high intensity nature of these workouts increase overall metabolic function far and above the low intensity workouts, and keeps it raised for up to 48hours following the session. This is especially apparent when it comes to improving insulin sensitivity. This is why I like it so much, and if I was forced to pick one over the other, it would be HIIT style routines for this very reason.

So just clarity, a HIIT style workout will include full body weight training incorporating large compound style movements such as squats, leg press, dead-lifts, chest press, shoulder press and seated rows. These movements recruit the largest muscle groups in the body to maximize this metabolic response. HIIT can also include interval workouts such circuit training and sprint work. The key is performing cyclical bursts of intense activity, followed by a rest and recovery period I.e. a 10 second hill sprint, followed by a 30 second walk back to the starting point.

Your Plan of Action

Whatever camp you find yourself in, it's important to just get yourself moving. I like to cover all bases with my clients and see what works best for the individual after some time implementing the various methods. And of course their own lifestyle, work and family commitments and schedules will be factored into this too.

However, the following is an overview of what I like to start out with. A base template I will prescribe for a typical week in terms of a workout program to reduce insulin resistance. It takes advantage of the body's natural hormonal fluctuations and rhythms. Insulin sensitivity is typically elevated in the morning, so more prolonged low intensity workouts will be performed here for instance.

However, once this natural sensitivity wears off at around 3pm, then it's time to employ the HIIT style sessions. This will artificially prompt another insulin sensitivity spike within the system, stimulating the skeletal muscles to uptake more blood glucose than they ordinarily would at this time, and store it in the form of muscle glycogen.

This is a clever trick you can play on the body in order to more efficiently regulate blood sugar levels. And as I say, this increased metabolic effect can last for up to two days depending on just how hard you worked yourself.

So here is my suggestion on how to structure your workouts on a daily basis. How to split up your sessions and the advancements you can make from week-to-week or month-to-month, once your overall fitness levels and conditioning improves:

Beginner/Low Fitness Level

AM - 20 minutes of light walking/cycling or swimming (Every other day)

PM - 30 minute full body resistance or sprint/interval workout (3 times a week)

Intermediate/Moderate Fitness Level

AM - 30 minutes of moderate walking/cycling or swimming (5 times a week)

PM - 45 minute full body resistance or sprint/interval workout (4 times a week)

Advanced/High Fitness Level

AM - 45 minutes of moderate walking/cycling or swimming
(Every day)

PM - 1 hour full body resistance or sprint/interval workout
(5 times a week)

*Note: Never perform more than three full body resistance workouts a week. This style of weight training can tax the central nervous system heavily, so you want to make sure you can recover. This really only comes into play for the advanced level individuals who are performing 5 HIIT sessions a week. So at most do 3 full body resistance workouts combined with 2 sprint/interval sessions per week.

Of course this is simply a guideline to follow, what has worked best for me and my clients over the years. However, any workout routine should be tailored towards the individual as much as possible. If you want to enlist the help of an experienced and qualified personal trainer within your local gym than do so. They will be able to better guide you through a more specialized program, and give you the added motivation to stick with it. My aim here is to simply give you an overview and outline to help get you started. So what are you waiting for!

Things to keep in mind

Once again, always ensure that you are eating enough and sticking to your meal plans. As we have already seen, metabolic damage can occur just as easily when taxing the body too heavily without adequate nutrition to fuel this activity. In this sense, keep the intense resistance and HIIT style workouts until the afternoon, when you have fully replenished your muscle glycogen stores.

In reality, any form of psychical activity, whether that be moderate cardio style exercise or intense weight training, will improve insulin sensitivity and reduce blood cholesterol and harmful lipid levels. So you simply have to get yourself to the gym. If you aren't already a member of one, then go sign up!

As with any lifestyle or positive behavioral change, consistency is the key. So build this into your routine as a daily habit and the results will start taking care of themselves. And of course, if you have any health concerns regarding physical activity and exercise, you should always consult your doctor before taking on such a program. The above is just an outline with regards to what is typically safe and beneficial for the average and healthy individual with slight insulin resistance.

BONUS CHAPTER

(From "Sugar Detox : A Nutritionists Guide")

CHAPTER 7: DRINKS & BEVERAGES - THE EASIEST WAY TO REDUCE YOUR SUGAR INTAKE

My original intention was to simply add this section on drinks & beverages within the previous chapter with the sugar free meal plans. However, over the years I have come to realize how important a persons beverage choice is with regards to reducing sugar & weight loss for that matter. It really is the low hanging fruit when its comes to cutting out the sweet stuff from your diet.

In truth, most folks simply do not realize just how much added sugar their favorite drinks contain. This is especially true when it comes to soda's. A regular coke (12 ounce can) contains 39 grams of sugar! The situation is similar for just about every soda brand on the market. I'm not simply trying to single out Coke here. Even iced lemon tea's contain a lot of added sugar unless you ask for none!

It's literally everywhere. Ever thought that buying that "healthy" sports or isotonic drink is the answer? Think again. I actually spent a few semesters studying the contents of these beverages during my undergraduate. They are all essentially made up from a mixture of the following three components, just in varying quantities. They do of course contain some artificial flavorings and other additives, but the big three are:

- Water - The base fluid for the drink.

- Sodium - To aid in retaining the water for hydration.

- Glucose - Yes sugar! For energy.

Now depending on the brand I.e. Gatorade, Lucozade etc and also the climate the specific drink was designed for (yes these are designed for athletes!). These factors will play a big role in the amounts of the above three components found in these bottles.

For example, drinks intended for those competing in hotter and more humid climates, will contain higher water and sodium levels as its more important to remain hydrated during these conditions above all else. The sodium actually tricks the kidneys into thinking that you are less hydrated than you actually are, so decides to retain more fluid in the body than it otherwise would. Clever right.

However, those drinks designed for cooler climates typically contain a higher percentage of glucose, as hydration is less of an issue. In this case the extra energy source is given precedence over hydration. So keep this in mind the next time you are feeling sporty and reach for one of the colorful "health" drinks in the supermarket fridge.

If you haven't just completed a 10k run or mammoth workout, or plan on doing so in the next 30 minutes… then put it back. In fact, sugar consumption around training times is one of the only times I believe it to be allowable. This is due to the body being about to burn these carbs off as energy substrates. Or replacing the liver and muscle glycogen you have just worked off post workout. Again, I talk in greater detail regarding general carbohydrate timing within "Intermittent Fasting: A Nutritionists Guide".

However in general, the regular person should simply cut out all of the above sugary beverage choices. Especially when initially attempting a sugar detox. Instead, replace these drinks with any combination of the following alternatives and you will notice a big difference in your weight and overall health as a result.

Healthier Sugar Free Alternatives

Water!

For most people, simply replacing every drink they consume with a glass of water, would literally halve their daily sugar intake. It would also provide them no end of additional health benefits such as clearer skin, better concentration and improved sleep etc. All this coming from elevated hydration levels. However, I realize this isn't always feasible as people do require some variance to stay the course.

Herbal, Green, Peppermint Tea (no sugar)

My most effective method of performing a sugar detox is with herbal teas. They are light on the stomach, taste great and give you a little caffeine boost to boot. Try not to overdo these. But if you feel yourself becoming tired or fatigued, especially during the afternoon, make yourself a cup of your favorite tea which should get you through until your next meal.

Black Coffee (no sugar)

If the herbal teas are not doing it for you, you have one more ace card up your sleeve. That is a strong coffee. Avoid sugar laden cappuccinos and the like. A strong black coffee should give you a large enough caffeine hit to squash any significant carb cravings. I know this is simply swapping one vice for another. But in the beginning stage of a sugar detox you have to do what you can to stay the course. Just fix one thing at a time!

Other Drinks to Avoid

Fruit Juices

You need to be cautious when it comes to juices. You have to be cognizant of your natural sugar intake for the day. I usually recommend no more than 2-3 servings of fruit per day during the first few weeks of detoxing. So one freshly pressed orange juice a day isn't an issue. But avoid cartoned fruit juices at all cost. They contain so much added sugar it almost puts them on par with full fat soda's!

On the days you are having fruit for breakfast or a smoothie, definitely refrain from any homemade juices and stick to water and tea that day.

Diet Drinks

Also avoid "diet" drinks and "zero sugar" beverages as they contain a lot of artificial sweeteners, such as aspartame & stevia, which are almost as bad as their full sugar counterparts. Studies have found that they may even promote weight gain to a similar degree compared with their sugar alternatives, not to mention a potential increased cancer risk too.

I used to drink Coke Zero as I thought I could use the caffeine hit without the calories. But I now simply opt for the herbal tea or black coffee options if I really need a pick me up. I would suggest you do the same. If you really are used to drinking these drinks and want to switch to "diet" version to begin with, then do so. But transitioning off of them as quickly as possible is the wise move to make.

If you really experience intense sugar cravings than make yourself one of the herbal tea's or black coffee first up. Then wait 30 minutes. If you are still experiencing the hunger pangs, then go brush your teeth! This may seem like a weird thing to do in the middle of the day, but it serves a clever little mind trick.

Nobody wants to eat or drink sugary things when they have the fresh taste of toothpaste in their mouth. You will find that your cravings will naturally subside when doing this, or will at least get you through until your next sugar free meal time!